EAT
YOURSELF
TO
DEATH

Culina Salus

First published in Great Britain in 2007 by Perseverance Works

1

EAT YOURSELF TO DEATH

Culina Salus

THE OBESITY EPIDEMIC IS UPON US

How to prevent your food choices from killing you

"Unless you change how you are, you will always have what
you have got"
Jim Rohn

For Wambui,Kamau and Adora my beloved constant companions on the journey climbing mountains,struggling across deserts and walking through the valleys.

EAT YOURSELF TO DEATH

Culina Salus

People are actually being slowly poisoned by their food choices

"Death ain't nothing but a heartbeat away"

"Gangsters Paradise" Coolio

INGRIEDIENTS

Nothing good comes easy

Lets make it clear from the outset; there are no quick fixes to changing your food choices permanently. it will be difficult, you will have to make sacrifices, you will get depressed at your lack of progress ,you will bury your head in the sand, you will feel hopeless, you will fall off the wagon, you will climb back on again, you will buy the wrong foods, you will succumb to the takeaway temptation, you will devour a meal for two and wash it down with enough fizzy soft drink to float a boat, you will squeeze into your clothes, you will delude yourself that you are losing fat but all you have lost is water, you will not be able to see certain parts of your body, unless you look in a large mirror, you will take part in every diet craze going, you will wonder, how the fuck, did I get this big? You will ask your partner; does my bum look big in this? You will comfort eat, you will throw up, you will not be able to look at yourself in the mirror.

You will do all of the above and more but if you persist with the ideas outlined in this book, you will triumph. It will be a bloody hard battle but in the words of Winston Churchill; "never give in, never, never, never".

Nec aspera terrent

Change begins when you decide to do something about your food choices and your lifestyle.
Make a decision to change for the better.
Then stick with it.

The choices you make, not the circumstances you find yourself in, will determine your success.

IT TAKES A NATION OF MILLIONS…….

In the United Kingdom:
Population: 60 million plus

11 million men over weight

9 million women over weight

12 million men and women obese

2 million overweight school children

Britons; the fattest people in Europe

By the time ,you read this the numbers above, would have sadly increased

Eat yourself to life.
IT'S a simple message really, if you refuse to change your eating poor habits, you will eventually eat yourself to death, too dramatic?
The world health organisation reports that obesity is a world wide epidemic and is estimated to cause 9000 deaths, annually in the United Kingdom alone. Britons are the fattest people in Europe, costing the National Health Service over £1 billion every year. Being obese can send you to a premature grave. The top 3 takers of life in the western world; heart disease, cancers and stroke can be directly linked to our food choices, a deadly side effect of our affluent societies.
Poor eating habits will lead to increased weight, which will turn into obesity, leading to increased risk of: heart disease, many forms of cancer such as breast, liver, uterus and colon, Stroke, High blood pressure, Kidney stones, Asthma, Depression (*every*

time you see your reflection and think about your uncontrolled eating) Diabetes, Infertility, Gall bladder disease, Osteoarthritis, Sleep apnea (*your excess weight causes you to stop breathing*)

Death by food
You know deep inside your heart that the junk you are eating is ruining your health. That thought flashes in your mind every time, you go shopping for clothes, for food, every time you look in the mirror or stand on the scales, every time you eat another chocolate bar, or order that extra large pizza or order your fourth takeaway meal of the week. You know that you are killing yourself slowly, bite by bite, munch by munch, burger-by-burger, cake-by-cake, fizzy drink by fizzy drink. You are slowly eating yourself to death.

There are no new facts in this book, no new research to report, no new diet fad to promote, the recommendations outlined here have been suggested and presented countless times in a million different places. This is a fat free, lean version of all the information, you need to live longer. You don't need to wade through facts and figures in a two hundred page book to get the information that you need. This book is a short, quick reminder of what you need to know and do to help yourself.

Yes, you must help yourself, the reason for the epidemic of excess weight is that we eat far too much high calorie food, overdosed with sugar and fat and don't burn it off with enough physical activity.

Whose fault is it? Fast food outlets? the food industry? Supermarkets? Feckless governments? You can blame all of the above but the person in the mirror must take the major share of the blame.

In these days of compensation culture, every one knows their rights but personal responsibility has crawled down a hole and died.

Eat what is in front if you
Take responsibility for your own actions and remember that, if you have children, you are their parent and not their friend. Many parents are quite feckless when it comes to their children's food choices. They no longer possess the gumption to make their children eat, what is in front of them. Giving children control of what goes in the shopping basket is wrong. Choice does not benefit children, they tend to become fussy eaters and veer towards sugary and fatty foods, Parents have abdicated their responsibility to provide good nutrition for their children, as a result these days you think children were the ones who went to work, earned the wages and decided what food shopping had to be done .

HOW many of these diets have you tried?
Slim fast
Mayo clinic
Warrior
Apple cider vinegar
Sonoma
Optimal
Glycaemic index
Beverly hills
Israel army
Herbalife
Liquid
Cabbage soup
Grapefruit
Makers
Zone
South beach
Scarsdale
Atkins

Jenny Craig
Blood type
Pritikin
Ornish
F Plan
Maple syrup
Hay
Protein power
Nutrisystem
Rosedale
Macrobiotic
Hip and thigh
Peanut butter
Hamptons
Cambridge
Purple
Neanderthin

Diets
Do
Not
Work
Let's get that damn straight!
95% of people who go on a diet have within two years, piled the weight and then some back on.

"There are no short cuts to any place worth going" Beverly Sills

It took you a long time to grow as large as you have, it will also take you a long time to lose the fat, but the greater your focus and corresponding actions on losing weight, the quicker it will disappear

Change what you eat

Cut the crap!

Compos sui

Discipline, will power and shopping list required

Interlude

Talking about a revolution

"No real social change has ever been brought about without a revolution, revolution is but thought carried into action"

Emma Goldman

2007; The norm is slim
The exception is overweight

2020; The norm is overweight
The exception is slim

Is it time for change,or do we just carry on munching ourselves to death?

End of interlude

The food industry will never stop creating addictive health ruining delights; it is what they were created to do. Junk food is profitable and sells extremely well.
You will have to become a rebel, start a revolution, and refuse to be a dumping ground for their products. Tell the food industry to go fuck itself by boycotting their lethal products and aggressively lobby them to produce decent

quality food.

The food industry is populated by the amoral who with the cooperation of the weak government you elected will sell you products that will trash your health.

The government cannot come to our rescue, it is under pressure from its paymasters, the food industry to ease, delay and soften any new restrictions, which may curb their profits.

Action speaks louder than words

FAST FOOD IS SLOW POISON
STOP BUYING JUNK FOOD

JUNK food has high levels of fat, salt, sugar and additives, making it energy dense, but it is almost completely devoid of vitamins and fibre. Advances in food technology, has allowed the food industry to churn out junk food in greater amounts and varieties. This junk is cheap to manufacture and has a long shelf life, this has made junk food the darlings of the food industry and supermarkets as they give greater profit margins.

The devourer behind all this is the junk food loving public who consumes ever increasing amounts of this *faux* food.

Why let someone else determine what goes into your body, you would never let a stranger into your home to dump garbage, so why do you allow scientists determine what you eat. The majority of what we eat is designed and created in laboratories, mother nature has been shackled and made to do man's will for example, strawberries grown in plastic tunnels all year round, chickens bred to be devoid of feathers, giant genetically modified salmon or the monstrous looking Belgian blue double muscled cattle specially bred to produce lean meat. Products created to increase profits and necessary to benefit your health. Why do you continue to pour chemical concoctions down your families' throats, how much cola do you really need to drink? A soft drink that will clean a copper coin or dissolve a tooth; is this the stuff you want to drink in large quantities on a daily basis?

Why give your child a glass of water, which contains six teaspoons of sugar, with added colouring, phosphoric acid, and artificial sweeteners? You might think it's harmless but it is wise?

Avoid processed food products and keep to real food, plant based food, the further a product is removed from its natural state, the more likely, it will contain a plethora of additives, fat, sugar and salt, the less items on the label the better. (Caveat emptor, not all items are legally required to be put on the label)

Good food is a meal that you plan, buy ingredients, prepare, cook and enjoy. The cheapest prepared meals tend to be packed with sugar, fat, salt and white flour, which makes them extremely tasty and addictive, but the added sugar and salt give a satisfying mouth feel and that should not be confused for taste.

Salty and sugary snacks such as crisps, cakes and chocolates are not food substitutes; they are what used to be called "in-betweens", something to tide you over, between proper nutritious meals. These snacks are "treats" something you had once in a fucking blue moon, NOT everyday on the way to work, at work, at your lunch break, when you are bored, on the way home. The rarity has become common, at the expense of our health and physical well-being

The cash rich,time poor myth

A marketing wizard and a scientist conjures up an "on the go" breakfast cereal and milk bar and sell you the idea that this sugar laden, fat saturated mixture from hell is a substitute for a proper breakfast for you and your kids, and you brought into this idea. Really! Have we become so gullible?

The food advertising industry has managed to convince everybody that due to our busy lifestyles, we no longer have the time to prepare our food, we are far too busy living to get cooking, we have swallowed this idea completely and have abdicated the responsibility of our basic healthy nutrition to scientists and marketing firms, allowing them to feed us any unholy concoction that they like, as long as it is profitable, they will sell it to us regardless of any adverse side effects. As they say "caveat emptor"

We have the ability to make time for everything else but the food industry has successfully convinced us that we do not have time to cook, the number one activity, that will bring the greatest health benefits to our lives. They have taken on the mantle to free us from the tyrannical grip of the kitchen by providing us with meal solutions for every situation.

People now spend more time choosing their clothes, new car, holiday, and celebrity gossip magazines than on what they eat.

We consume without question everything the food industry, supermarkets and takeaways send our way. We hardly question, how our food is grown? what is added to it ?, where it is flown in from ?, what it contains ?, what the food manufacturers do not have to put on the label ?

We are on a non-stop, unthinking feast, hell! We are no better than a docile cow taken out to graze on a field; just eating, shitting, not asking questions, eat more, shit and the cycle never ends.

WAKE UP!

OUR food is killing us slowly, and that is the issue, we give the least attention to. We purchase food with our eyes, focusing on how it looks, its size, its packaging, is it appealing? Attractive? sexy? Every other important consideration has been rescinded. Our relationship with food has been warped by our laziness and the marketing departments of the supermarkets and food manufacturers, in the past our relationship could be described as follows:

Farm to shops (*mainly independent grocers, butchers not many supermarkets*) to kitchen to dinner table

The present could be seen as:

Farm or laboratory to supermarkets (*very few grocers or butchers*) to kitchen or microwave to dining table or plate on lap in front of TV.

The future:

Laboratory to supermarket to microwave to plate on lap in front of TV

Homes of the future will not need a kitchen, just a shelf for the microwave, a bin for the prepared meals packages and a fridge freezer to store them.

Take control, help yourself, and make a change by cooking your own food.

To borrow a phrase *"can't cook, won't cook"* then if you can;

Learn to drive

Learn a new job

Learn a new skill

Plan a holiday

You can learn how to choose your ingredients, prepare and cook them. Switch off the great time stealer; television or if you can't do without it, record your favourite programme or put a television in the kitchen, get off the phone and cook yourself a healthy meal.

And if on first couple of tries, your creation gets burnt or tastes like cardboard, try, try, try again until you succeed.

If we continue to increase our consumption of prepared meals, then a few decades, there will not be any need for fresh produce, no exotic ingredients, no condiments, who will need them? You can't cook, your children sure as hell will never learn how to. Who will teach and encourage them? Schools junked cooking lessons long ago.

The only thing you can teach them is how to use the microwave, so they can say "mummy and daddy taught us how to open a packet and nuke it in a microwave!". All you have done is create more customers for the chilled food industry. So why the fuck, would anybody need to sell ingredients when it is more convenient and much more profitable to add value and sell the finished product.

Pop into supermarkets like Iceland or Farm-foods, nary a fresh product will you find, no bits and pieces, just the finished product, all you have to do is apply heat. Doesn't the future taste tempting!

MAKE A CHANGE

It all begins with what you put in your shopping basket, simply don't buy the junk and get the good healthy stuff instead like

Dried fruit instead of sweets

Nuts instead of crisps and biscuits

Wholegrain bread instead of white

Water instead of sugary soft drinks

Cooking from scratch, instead of prepared meals.

Fuck all the ads you have seen, it is far more appealing to assemble ingredients and prepare a meal than to pop a ready meal packaged by poorly paid staff in a suspect factory into a microwave.

You say "I love my food" but your long term heath is being destroyed by this love affair

Food for thought

Go into a fried chicken, Chinese or Indian takeaway outlet, and observe the staff serving, they are not overweight or even fat; it is plainly obvious they do not consume the food

they are selling you. Maybe they know something you don't.

Because you don't drink

Because you don't smoke

Because you think that you don't have any vices
Does not mean that you have to give yourself permission to eat the wrong things

You will end up dying at the same as the smoking alcoholic.

Interlude

Quis custodiet ipsos custodie

Who is watching out for consumer health? Do you trust the government, food industry or supermarkets to watch out for your health? Have you put your unwavering faith in them to ensure that the food supply is completely safe, if so who is watching them. Modern society runs on money, international conglomerates have a turnover of billions from selling food to us; they also spend billions advertising their wares to us.

There is very little money being spent on information to inform us that our food choices are killing us. Who is on our side? Who is protecting our health?

The democratically elected government? That system which is greatly influenced by lobbyists, representing the highly influential food industry, the system that has political parties funded by donations from "Big business". With this system dominating the western world can you ever imagine the government ever biting the hand that literally feeds it?

The same government that prevents the food industry from lying to us but allows them to be economical with the truth, with food labels, for example contents do not have be on label as long as they fall within the minimum legal amounts.

The same government that funds a study into food additives that proves they have a detrimental effect on children's health but will still not ban them.

So who is watching those who are supposed to watch over us?

End of interlude.

Revive the appetiser

Start me up!

Ab actu ad posse valet illation

Discipline, willpower and starter required
Revive the appetiser
IT'S a simple trick really; fill yourself up partly with a starter before you gorge yourself on the main course. It is back to basics; starter, main course, dessert or "afters" as they were once called. It could be the following:
A large glass of water
A piece of fruit or fruit cocktail (an apple before a meal is known to keep one regular)
Low calorie soup
Small salad
A glass of vegetable juice
A starter will help dampen your appetite, but you should choose a healthy starter, 2 slices of garlic bread before a 12 inch pizza is not a healthy starter, a large of glass of water, apple or bowl of chicken noodle soup will reduce the amount of the main meal, you plan to eat. It is a great method to use to gradually reduce and wean yourself off eating large amounts of food. It's as simple as eating a chocolate bar, fill yourself up a low or zero calorie starter to reduce the amount of high calories consumed. It will also help you meet your 5 daily portions of fruit and vegetables.

"All things being equal, the simplest solution tends to be the right one"
 Occam's razor

Interlude

We have never

We have never had a protest march onto the houses of parliament, to demand that our government, regulate the food industry till their pips squeak

We have never carried out a boycott of crappy junk food, forcing manufacturers to provide healthy food.

We have never thought that our food was too cheap and be willing to pay more for better quality. In the food industry, the maxim, you pay for what you get, has never been truer.

We have never seriously demanded to know why our government has sold off playing fields

We have never asked why there are hardly any police *walking* the streets, as a result many parents feel that the streets are unsafe, so we keep our children indoors, watching television, playing computer games, denying them the freedom to run about till they are breathless.

We have never learnt how to cook, so we are completely reliant on health destroying prepared meals. You cannot cook, you child will never learn how to, you do not need a crystal ball to realise that their food choices will be completely controlled by others.

All the food industry needs to completely control our food choices, is for people to remain silent and do nothing. Complaining about food additives, sugar and salt levels in food is not action. The food industry merely acknowledges our complaints but does not swerve from its path of totally controlling our food choices.

End of interlude

Two litres of water daily

Get a drink habit!

Exitus acta probat

Discipline, willpower and a bottle required

"If you flavour water, it's a soft drink"

George Carlin

Water, water, water everywhere

THE earth is covered by 70% of water
The body is comprised of 60% water
The human brain is 85% water
The lungs are 90% water
Blood is 83% water
Muscles are 70% water
Bones are 25% water

It is obviously better to rehydrate yourself with the stuff you are made from, yet we drink so little of it in its pure form, the real thing, plain water, not flavoured, not fortified, not a hint flavoured versions of water that tend to be high in calories or sugar substitutes. Drinks containing caffeine will leech, water out of your system, making you dehydrated. If you are dehydrated, your blood has lower water content, making your circulation sluggish, your brain less active, you can't concentrate and feel tired.

Why drink more water?

It moisturizers your skin, helps you hydrate your body, keeps your body system working efficiently such as digestion, controlling temperature and helps transports waste materials, making bowel movements softer and easier to pass.

It flushes toxins out of your system, helps kidneys and liver function properly, and helps avoid bladder and urinary tract infections.

Helps control a fever, replaces moisture lost to sweating and will thin out mucus.

Increases your metabolism and energy levels

Drink two litres of pure water daily, quite an easy feat to achieve, if you put your mind to it, start your day at home or work with a 2 litre jug or bottle and make your aim to finish it at set time, for example at work make sure you finish it by the time you go home.

Another method to get more fluid into your body is to consume more fruit and vegetables, as they are mainly comprised of water.

Water is the only drinking liquid on this planet that is completely harmless.

Tea and coffee contains caffeine

Milk is fattening, some people, are lactose intolerant

Soft drinks, fruit juices: sugary and down right dangerous

Beer, spirits and wine; use with care

Reasons to Drink Water*

Water is absolutely essential to the human body's survival. A person can live for about a month without food, but only about a week without water.

Water helps to maintain healthy body weight by increasing metabolism and regulating appetite.

Water leads to increased energy levels. The most common cause of daytime fatigue is actually mild dehydration.

Drinking adequate amounts of water can decrease the risk of certain types of cancers, including colon cancer, bladder cancer, and breast cancer.

For a majority of sufferers, drinking water can significantly reduce joint and/or back pain.

Water leads to overall greater health by flushing out wastes and bacteria that can cause disease.

Water can prevent and alleviate headaches.

Water naturally moisturizes skin and ensures proper cellular formation underneath layers of skin to give it a healthy, glowing appearance.

Water aids in the digestion process and prevents constipation.

Water is the primary mode of transportation for all nutrients in the body and is essential for proper circulation.

*Source All About Water.org

"Water is life's matter and matrix, mother and medium. There is no life without water"
Albert Szent-Gyorgyi

Interlude part 1

Your focus determines your reality
PEOPLE will spend all day at work, thinking and talking about what they will have for dinner, they will chat obsessively about the chips and chicken dippers meal they are going have that evening: fatcrap.
Focus on eating fatcrap food, and you will spread like a balloon filled with air, focus on a dinner of grilled chicken breast with green salad tossed in a low calorie balsamic dressing, with a fresh fruit cocktail to follow, what do you think, will eventually happen?

After all you are what you eat

Formula for success in the chilled food industry:
Food ingredients sold separately are not very profitable, but combine them into a ready chilled meal hence adding value; you have now created a very profitable product. How do you achieve sales revenue in the billions? By convincing people that they are too busy too cook and cooking is a hassle, and you have provided them with a convenient alternative. With your partner, the ubiquitous supermarkets and an advertising budget in the billions and after a couple of decades, your campaign has been so successful that your customers are completely reliant on you and have abandoned the kitchen. They cannot cook and their children cannot even boil an egg, you have successfully created another generation for your products.

Iinterlude part 2

Science; a moveable feast
SCIENCE is not a fact; it is a prevailing theory that has not been disproved and discarded.
Because it's safe to eat
Because it's not harmful
Because it has no proven side effects
Because there is no conclusive evidence of it causing...... (*Finish the sentence yourself*)

Because it has been passed by the dept of.... (*Finish the sentence yourself*) does not mean that it is good for you.

Science created hydrogenated edible oils, which we all assumed was safe, since men in white coats wearing glasses had created it, we consumed products containing and fried in hydrogenated oil until another bunch of yahoo's moved the goal posts and told us that trans fats, a by product of hydrogenated oils was actually harmful to our health. Science created additives such as tartrazine, sunset yellow, carmoisine and sodium benzoate that were once widely regarded as safe and legal have now been declared by scientists as detrimental to health, while many people have been campaigning for years that these additives were not safe, scientists regarded their experience as "anecdotal" which means you are talking crap that cannot be proved by science.

Question; science and food should not mix; agree or disagree?

End of interludes

Avoid the fearsome four

The usual suspects;
Sugar, salt, fat and white flour

Veritas vos liberabit

Willpower, discipline and abstinence required

To lengthen thy life, Lessen thy meals

Benjamin Franklin

What's your poison?
Food's made from white flour, salt, sugar and fat are junk food or what we call fatcrap, the perverse thing about fatcrap is that it tastes good. the taste sensations of salt, sugar and fat are so instinctive and addictive, they can never be fully satisfied, that's why one doughnut, one cookie, one piece of fried chicken, one chocolate bar is never enough.

Interlude

Ode to fatcrap
Fatcrap; super convenient
Fatcrap: destroyer of health and life
Fatcrap; high in calories
Fatcrap; quick to prepare
Fatcrap; slow to kill
Fatcrap; turns people into balloons
Fatcrap; tastes good
Taste good; get fat
Taste good; get cancer
Taste good; get ill
Taste good; can't run, walk or climb stairs

Taste good; no stamina hence 2 minute sex minithon
Taste good; get diabetes
Taste good; clothes don't fit
Taste good; very slow poison
Taste good; fat children

Too dramatic, over the top, then why are millions of people on a diet or watching their weight and what they eat? Because they know that cemeteries are being rapidly being filled up by people who have eaten themselves to death.

End of interlude

FAT: THE WORLDS MOST WANTED
Naturally saturated fat raises your blood cholesterol, saturated fat can be found in meat, milk and milk products such cheese and butter but most of the fat we consume are
artificially produced trans fatty acids such as hydrogenated fats, this is the process where vegetable oil is heated, hydrogen gas added, creating hydrogenated oil, which is a source of trans fats.
They are mainly used to prolong the shelf life of products like crisps, biscuits and other baked products, it has been reported that these trans fats, are absorbed into the brain, displacing healthy fats, reducing the brains ability to transmit messages between cells.
Trans fats have been banned in New York and Denmark, companies such as KFC, McDonald's, Starbucks have banned then as well. The most important thing is not that these items have been banned but the fact that we have been consuming these products for years.
Dangers of too much fat:
A high fat diet can lead to breast cancer

Calorie overload as fat contains twice the number of calories of a similar amount of protein or carbohydrates

Excess fat can increase the risk of fertility problems

Excess fat leads to obesity

Excess fat causes heart disease

Fat causes some forms of cancer

Excess fat causes diabetes

Excess fat causes high blood pressure

Excess fat kills

Some fat is good is good for health, it supplies energy, helps absorb vitamins and essential fatty acids such as omega 3 are beneficial to health and well being, especially to children.

Use good oils such as olive oil, sesame oil, groundnut oil, flax seed oil, corn oil and sunflower oil

In the long term:

Reduce all fat intake

Greatly reduce the consumption of processed food and snacks

Read food labels, to help you make the right choices

Eat food close to its original state, such as fruit, nuts, vegetables etc if you cannot tell the original source of food, avoid.

Chose low fat products, also lean meats, fish and chicken and most importantly:

Cook your own food

White flour:colour me badd

THERE is nothing good in white flour, it is truly devoid of any redeeming qualities, mainly as a result of the fibre, the nutritious wheat germ and essential vitamins and minerals like chromium, which helps keep blood sugar levels stable, have been lost in the refining process. A similar process also happens with white rice; all rice is grown brown and is then polished white. Now fibreless white flour (and rice) becomes compacted as they pass through the system, causing constipation.

Also during the refining process, white flour is aged with chlorine dioxide, then chalk and ammonium carbonate and alum are added to "improve" it. Then this product of nature, improved by man, is turned into bread, burger buns, pitta bread, pizza bases, cakes, biscuits, doughnuts, and numerous pastry products; all visually pleasing and tasty products but full of empty calories.

Interlude

Become a food luddite

Can technology improve upon Mother Nature? The most beneficial foods for healthy living are still in their natural state or quite close to it. Nuts, seeds, whole grains, pulses, fruits, vegetables, leafy greens, jacket potatoes, lean meat, grilled chicken, fish compare this to foods such as cakes, chocolates, crisps ,burgers, chicken nuggets, pizza, cookies, biscuits, items so far removed from their original state that you would never imagine that the aforementioned nuggets came from a chicken.

Man and technology can and has improved lives in health care, safety, communications, people live longer, millions own personal computers, mobile phones, cars are safer but industrialization has not brought corresponding health benefits to the food, we consume, we produce more food with the help of fertilizers, additives, chemicals, intensive farming and mechanization but all this technology has made food plentiful and cheap but it has made us unhealthy, over-weight, obese, diabetic, hyperactive, moody, greedy, gluttonous, cancerous, cheap, unappreciative and aggressive. This particularly unholy combination of food and technology is ruining people's health and sending thousands to an early grave.

If aliens ever wanted to take over this planet all they would have to do is send us the technology to produce tasty, fatty, sugary and salty fatcrap and in a few decades, half of the world's population would have eaten themselves to death, the surviving half would be too fat to fight, making global conquest easier.

Maybe its all ready happened? After all it would take a truly alien frame of thinking to feed cows, with meat and bone meal from the carcasses of cattle and sheep as a protein supplement, leading to mad cow disease. After all humans know that from beginning of time, cattle have been herbivores.

End of interlude

Sugar; hard habit to break

Sugar is the most addictive substance on earth, many have managed to wean themselves off drugs, alcohol and cigarettes but sugar is the hardest habit to break, an exaggeration? Just try to go cold turkey off sugar and all artificial sweeteners for 30 days. Don't forget the hidden sugar in foods such as burger buns, cooking sauces. Since we can live without refined sugar, then any amount, we consume has no beneficial effect to our health, then to consume mass quantities of sugar is to invite ill heath.

Any food item with more than 15 grams of sugar per 100 grams has high sugar content.

Why is sugar public enemy number one?

It can suppress the immune system

It can cause hyperactivity, crankiness and difficulty in children

It can lead to cancer of the breast, ovaries, prostrate and rectum

It can cause tooth decay

It contributes to obesity

It can assist the growth of yeast infections, such as candida. Bacteria and yeast in our system feeds on sugar, too much and they multiply and weaken the immune system.

It can cause heart disease

It can increase cholesterol

It can contribute to diabetes

It feeds cancer

It kills the appetite, mama used to say "no sweets before your meal" as sugar dampens hunger pangs, making you eat less of the nutritious meal, mama had cooked, these days, mama is having a sugar rush herself, having overdosed on cakes, chocolates and fizzy drinks, all she is capable of doing is taking her kids down to the nearest fatcrap palace for a meal saturated with sugar, salt and fat.

Consuming too much sugar affects your skin, making you look old. its called glycation, sugar sticks to protein, hence making body tissues and organs lose elasticity, and since your skin is the body's largest organ, so the more sugar you consume equals increased glycation, equals faster aging, so whatever your true age, you look ten years older.

How does so much sugar get into our system? giving us permanent lust for sugar.

Millions of people are addicted to sugar, especially children, so food manufacturers put it into a large number of products, either in the form of sugar or cheap fructose sugar from corn, so you find sugar in products that would not have it, if you made the stuff yourself, like baked beans, cooking sauces (you have to keep stirring them to prevent the sugar from burning at the bottom of the pot) peanut butter, mayonnaise, ketchup, soups such as tomato, barbeque sauce, sweet chilli sauce. It is also a preservative, giving longer shelf.

A large amount of sugar we consume comes from

carbohydrates. All carbohydrates turn into sugar after you consume them, there are two types of carbohydrates; simple and complex

Simple or refined carbohydrates are high glycaemic index (GI) foods such as white flour, white rice, sugar, which turn into sugar in your blood stream, making your blood sugar level to rise quickly, which cause your body to produce insulin. Sending your blood sugar into a roller coaster drive of highs and lows, which makes you fatigued, exhausted, irritable and can cause headaches and migraines.

Insulin will bring down blood sugar levels but a side effect is that insulin quickens the transformation of calories into fat, which is stored in your most idle body regions such as the belly, bum, breasts and thighs as a result you gain weight, become obese, leading to diabetes or heart disease.

Complex carbohydrates tend to be low GI foods such as whole wheat, whole grains, fruits, vegetables and bananas are rich in fibre, which take longer for the body to absorb, as a result blood sugar rises very slowly, so there is no need for an insulin reaction.

This sweet temptress has many names such as molasses, corn syrup, dextrose, fructose, glucose, maltose, sucrose, corn sugar, invert sugar, lactose, levlose and milk sugar but underneath all those fancy names, she is still SUGAR!

Sugar is bad, bad, bad, bad, bad, bad, bad, bad, Bad, bad, bad, bad, bad, bad, bad, bad, bad, Bad, bad, bad, bad, bad, bad, bad, bad, bad, Bad, bad, bad, bad, bad, bad, bad, bad, bad, Bad, bad, bad, bad, bad,

bad, bad, bad, bad, Bad, bad, bad, bad, Bad, bad, bad, bad,

Bad, bad, bad, bad, bad, bad, bad, bad, bad, bad, bad, bad, bad, bad, Bad, bad, bad, bad, bad, bad, bad,

I'm sure you've got the point

SALT; Mad,bad and dangerous to consume

THE following is not breaking news; too much salt is bad for you, why:
It causes high blood pressure
It causes strokes
It causes heart attacks
It causes water retention
It worsens osteoporosis
It worsens asthma
It causes renal disease
It causes gastric cancer.
Most of the salt we consume, is found in processed foods, so to avoid it, you will need to cook your own food or read labels carefully.
How much is too much?
0.1 grams per 100 grams is low
0.2 to 0.4 grams 100 grams is medium
0.5 grams per 100 grams is high
The average consumption in the United Kingdom is 9.5grams per day.
You should not consume more than a total of 6 grams per day, so that single packet of ready salted

crisps (3.5 grams), you just ate, means that you are quickly filling up your daily quota.

Avoiding the bad boy

Do not sprinkle salt onto your food; do not forget that table sauces like ketchup, soy sauce, and items like burgers, ready meals and biscuits, contain large amounts of salt.

Reduce the amount of salt, stock cubes and bullion, you use in cooking, if you can, eliminate them completely, use more herbs, spices, lemons, limes, ginger, garlic and chillies, you will end up with tasty and not salty food.

Greatly reduce your intake of processed foods such as bread, baked beans, and breakfast cereals with high salt levels, sausages, salami, bacon, ham, hot dogs, soups, cheese, takeaways and ready prepared chilled or frozen meals.

Pop quiz?

Can you tell the difference between a salty food and a tasty food?

Interlude

Master reset

People will always default to convenient and easy habits, a lifestyle that ultimately makes them fat, lazy and wrecks their health. Habits such as:

Car driving instead of walking

Ready meals and takeaways instead of cooking

Watching television instead of cooking

Excuses instead of action

Buying special offers instead of sticking to your shopping list

Chocolates, crisps and cakes instead of fruit

Complaining instead of taking direct action

Acquiescence instead of revolution

Shopping instead of staging a boycott

master reset takes you back to a setting where events happen to you and shape your life, modern society contrives to make you a fat lazy docile consumer but a programmed planned life will make you different from everybody else, where you impress you will power upon events to create the life, you desire.

It is possible to eat what is good for you, to exercise on a regular basis, to question everything, to live your life according to your plan and not revert back to factory settings.

Lose your breath

Let's get physical

Mama used to say; move your lazy bones

Disce Pati

Discipline and will power definitely required
Move your mind and your ass will follow

Get busy one time
Regular exercise and physical activity has almost vanished from normal day to day activity, now, it is getting so bad, you really don't have to walk anywhere, you can work from home, do your banking online, pay bills by direct debit or online, all shopping can be done online, supermarkets will deliver to your home, takeaways will always oblige, rental movies are posted to you, so the only walking that you will ever do, is around the house. And if you have to go a little bit further, there is always the car. Assuming you steer clear of regular exercise, it is now possible that you can go for a whole year without ever getting out of breath, maybe for even longer. Can you remember the last time you were out of breath? When was the last time you walked for an hour, not counting the times you were stranded by the bus or train strikes and forced to walk.
Sexual activity has become two minute sessions, just before you run out of breath, as you no longer have the stamina to exert your body for any period of time.
If your claim to fame, is that you don't have time to exercise, then you must learn to multitask, if you can polish off a chicken tikka masala, whilst watching television, eating poppadums, drinking beer and sending a text on your mobile phone then you can sort yourself out by fitting activity into your lifestyle.

You have heard the following all before about the benefits of regular vigorous exercise; get a positive attitude, do something, do anything that increases your heart rate and leaves you breathless; wash the car, get moving, escape the couch, walk more, ditch the car, walk to school, climb the stairs, go to the gym, go for a run, go for a swim, go dancing, it greatly improves your health, it eases depression and stress, helps you live longer, get on your bike, make the time, kill the television, get a pedometer, vary the routine, walk during your lunch break, keeps you mentally sharp, take 10,000 steps daily, avoid the lift, set realistic goals, it increases energy levels, increases confidence in how your look, it will greatly benefit your kids, as they will copy your active lifestyle, reduces risk of heart disease, stroke and diabetes, run the marathon, exercise at home, start a walking club, mow the lawn, give it all you've got, power-walk, got trainers? Make sure they live up to their name, run to music, set yourself a goal, reward yourself when you achieve, exercise at the state of the art gym, exercise at the community centre, exercise at home, do gardening, do diy, get a personal trainer, become a personal trainer, walk the dog, jog with the dog, walk with your child, walk to school, never give up, just do it, be determined, prevents heart disease and stroke, reduces high blood pressure, reduces cholesterol, gives you time to think, reduces obesity, park further away from the supermarket main entrance, keep at it.
Exercise, you know it's good for you
Don't be ambitious, just get breathless
For God's sake do something
Your life depends on it

"I did not pay anybody to put on weight, so I'm sure not

going to pay anybody to lose it. I'm going to eat less and run, running is free and I will save money by eating less"

Mrs Ojo (On being advised to go to a gym)

THE MEANING OF LIFE:

Conceive your goals

Believe in yourself

Plan your work

Work your plan

Make the necessary sacrifices

Achieve your dream

Applies to everything you do, just do it.

Interlude

Eating dangerously
THE food industry will feed us with anything that has not been conclusively proven to be dodgy or harmful to our health. This situation normally continues until new research, which strongly suggests or proves that we have been eating dangerously, creates a health scare that is strongly backed by the public asking for change. Nothing will scare a company more into taking positive action than bad publicity.
Remember these food scares
Trans fats
Mono sodium glutamate
Saccharin
Artificial sweeteners such as aspartame
(The jury is still out)

Saturated fat
Salt levels in food
Pesticide residues on fruit and vegetables
Genetically modified foods
Sudan 1- potentially carcinogenic food dye
Para red- another carcinogenic food dye
Sodium benzoate- causes damage to DNA
Salmonella in fresh eggs
Antimony in bottled water
E.coli in salad vegetables
Sugary drinks causing pancreatic cancer
White bread causing cancer of the kidney
Growth hormones in beef causing cancer
Creutzfeldt jakob disease – popularly known as mad cow disease, mainly caused by feeding cattle with animal proteins.
All the above and more were once touted by the food industry as being safe to consume. It makes you wonder, what are you consuming
Now? That will turn out to be hazardous in the future

Food D I Y

Nothing good comes easy

Dimidium facti qui coepit habet

Willpower, discipline and acquiring cooking skills required

If you are too damn lazy or can't be bothered,to prepare and cook your own food,please stop reading,you have just waiting your time and money.(Thanks for buying the book anyway)

Repetition Is
The
Mother
Of
Skill -Tony Robbins

Food; do it yourself
Take your typical homemade shepherds pie, ingredients are lamb mince, onions, oil, herbs, spices, stock, salt, chopped tomatoes and mashed potatoes no more no less. Now go down and pick up a ready made version, read the ingredients list, check out the all additives.
Why so much crap in our foods? Preservatives to extend shelf life, added colours to improve appearance, and artificial flavours to heighten taste and restore aroma lost in the production process. Some of the usual suspects are aspartame, sodium benzoate, mono sodium glutamate, xanthan gum (used to bind food together, think reconstituted chicken nuggets) and the notorious E family.
Are you 100% SURE that continued consumption of

these substances will not do any long-term harm to your health? The food industry have repeated said their additives are safe, without any adverse side effects, with any industry worth billions of pounds at stake, would you really expect them to say any different? Some additives are made from coal tar, in a world where toilet waste is recycled into drinking water; we should not be surprised at the depths the food industry will sink to find a profit.

Why you should cook you own food;

You will reduce the amount of additives, you consume, it has been reported that people consume over 20 different additives daily

You know exactly what you put in your food

You will get to reduce and control the amount of fat, salt and sugar in your food.

You have complete control over your food choices

It's cheaper than buying chilled or frozen ready meals and you will get more value for your money.

Instead of a fatcrap ready meal which comes in various guises; chilled, frozen, takeaway, you get to prepare meals from scratch, grilling, steaming, baking using lean meat, chicken, fish, fruit and vegetables. Remember the days of well balanced "meat and two veg"

Your food will be fresher, with vitamins and minerals intact, which are essential for good health. A diet deficient of these, will affect the bodies' ability to fight of toxins, which can make your cells diseased and eventually cancerous.

Can't cook, won't cook, can't even boil water, you can learn.

If you have;

Learnt to drive

Learn a new language

Learn a new skill, new job, you can learn to cook

Can't cook?

Go to cookery classes, watch and learn from cookery

programmes, buy a cookbook, then practice till you come up with something edible then progress for there.

Won't cook?

Make the time, pre plan your meals, multitask, put a television in your kitchen, get off the telephone, put the mobile on voicemail, cancel that after work trip to the pub, start preparation the day before, start a cooking club with friends, cook meals and freeze them, schedule cooking time, take turns with your partner, get the kids to help, stop making excuses and being lazy, try out new recipes.

With the right amount of willpower, you can achieve the goal of cooking your meals.

Interlude

Numbers ruining the health of our children
2 Million Children are overweight
700,000 are obese
160,000 have high blood pressure
25% of girls and **20%** of boys are overweight
97% of 11 year olds do not get sufficient exercise
9 to **10** grams of salt per day is consumed by many children, well above the recommended daily limit of 6 grams
125 Kingsway,Aviation House, London WC2B 6NH : address of the Food Standards Agency, the feckless and ineffective government food watchdog that operates the regulation of the food industry for the benefit of business and not the consumer.
158 applications approved to dispose of playing fields since 1998
10 Downing St, London SW1A 2AA : address of the prime minister,start your million mum march for healthy food here.
70% of children drop out of sport after school
2 hours per week for physical activity set in the national curriculum
1 in 5 pupils do not get the minimum 2 hours

4 hours per day, the amount of television, your child has to watch daily to become obese

£587 million spent on food, soft drinks and fast food advertising in 2005

£143 million total budget for Food Standards Agency in 2006

£135 million total budget for Food Standards Agency in 2010

£7.357 billion: worth of the UK fast food sector in 2005, the largest in Europe, twice the size of Germany's and three times that of France

1000 plus scientists working in the chilled food industry

12000, the number of different chilled meals

80% of households in England buy ready meals

65% of lunch boxes contain unhealthy snack

31% of lunch boxes contain unhealthy drink

Our children may have to cope with all the above facts but determined, strong and focused parents have the power to nullify the effects of all the above on the children's health by making them move more, eating well and watching less television

Step up

Step on the scales Every darned day

Watch your weight

Semper Vigilans

Discipline and scale required
Watch the scales
Buy a scale preferably a digital one and weight yourself everyday and keep a record. The number displayed will tell you one of the following truths: exercise more, drastically reduce your portion size, cut out the fatcrap, it will also indicate weather you are on the right track to reaching your ideal weight or you have reached your goal.
Choose your target weight, with a date for achievement and work towards it by exercising, eating less and eating wisely and well. The scale will give an accurate impartial report on your progress.

How many bags are you carrying?
Lets say you are happen to be to be four stones overweight, which is approximately twenty five kilograms, which means in effect that you are carrying around with you twenty five bags of sugar(1 kg size),even being just two stone overweight is 12 kilograms,12 bags of sugar,12 bags of sugar, when you ;
Go shopping
Walk
Stand
Make love
Climb stairs

Run for the bus
Sleep
Run around with your kids
Head for the nearest fatcrap stall
Twenty four hours a day, carrying 12 fucking bags, it is any wonder? that your feet ache, your bad aches, your ankles ache, you hate how you look, you don't sleep well, always stressed, irritable, depressed, feel like crap, your clothes no longer fit.
It's those 12 damned bags. Lose them and you will feel better. I guarantee it. *Lose your excess luggage.*
Interlude

The talking scale

Talking scale says:

8 Stone; hello sexy

12 stone; love those curves

15 stone; what have you been eating?

17 stone; I'm struggling here

18 stone; GET OFF!

20 stone; GET THE FUCK OFF!

"Eat,drink and be morbidly obese"

Harold Faulkner

End of interlude

THE POWER OF SIX

The new black is 6

Nunquam non paratus

Willpower, discipline and preparation required

Never eat when you are hungry

Grazing is in

Eat small six meals daily as opposed to your one or two normal meal times. Why? This will stop you from feeling hungry, hence decreasing your food and calorie intake. It will also help you control your appetite.

It will stop your stomach bloating, from the strain of super size meals. So instead of 2 to 3 mountains to 6 small hills

These six mini meals ideally should be of your own making, they should be nutritious, helping you avoid salty, sugary and fatty alternatives.

Frequent meals will help you avoid the mid morning or afternoon dip, your alertness and energy levels will remain stable.

You will establish a regular eating pattern, hence sending signals to the body, that it is not being starved, so it does not need to store extra calories.

It will keep your system stimulated, making your metabolism burn more calories

It will help keep blood sugar stable

You may say why eat when you are not hungry, the whole point is to make sure that you do not get hungry, throw caution to the winds, pig out and eat yourself into a stupor.

Make sure that you never miss breakfast, wake up a little bit earlier or prepare the night before, this action alone will help your wallet, your life and help you steer clear of fat laden, chemical ridden, calorie busting, sugar over dosed and salt saturated purchases.

In case you didn't know, you don't have to eat everything you see, Learn to walk on by

Interlude

Question everything;trust no one

The advertisement proudly proclaims:

"Our range of food does not contain any artificial colourings, flavourings or additives"

The question you should be asking, are what are the sugar, salt and fat levels?

The label says;
Sugar free or No added sugar

The question you should be asking yourself is, although too much sugar consumption is down right deadly, it is still a natural product made from sugar beet or sugar cane, can the same be said of its artificial replacement, most likely to be aspartame.

Eat real food, not laboratory creations

EVERYDAY IS NOT CHRISTMAS(something mother used to say)

Mama also used to say; too much of anything is bad

Caveat emptor

Willpower and discipline required more than ever

Everything is for eating but everything is not for eating

You are allowed to say NO

Interlude

Dangerous habits

Dangerous habits 1
WHEN you open a packet of biscuits, do you:
1 Eat 2 or 3 and save the rest till next time
OR
2 Eat the whole 200 gram packet in one sitting

Number 2? You are in big trouble

Dangerous habits 2
The most deadly restaurant invention of recent times: "the all you can eat buffet" created for people who think quality and quantity are the same thing. First started by Indian restaurants, to increase trade on quiet Sundays. Now widely adopted and served everyday by Chinese restaurants and even some pizza restaurants. Buffet service removes all limitations, there are numerous dishes to choose from, so you feel obligated to try as many as possible, you make sure you do not leave the

restaurant, without making at least four trips to the food counter, probably changing plates every time to make you feel like its your first plate, besides you want to get your money's worth, in addition you have probably starved yourself before you got there, so you can wreck maximum damage on the buffet.

Its also accepted practice to be a glutton at a buffet, eating so much food that you can barely walk out of the restaurant.

Every day is not Christmas

Stop eating! Put down that burger, back away from the chocolate bar, you eat too much! All eating desires are met, what was once seasonal is now common place, available 365 days a year, for instance strawberry season in the United Kingdom is normally summer but why wait, when they can be flown in from all over the world, so strawberries are now available all year round in your local supermarket, never mind that they are tasteless, but at least you can indulge your strawberry addiction non stop.

People now eat and drink, everyday as if it was their final meal, on their last day on planet earth, every day is a Christmas dinner. Items once considered "treats" like soft drinks, cakes, chocolates are now being consumed as if they are going out of fashion. It's time to set up

Chocoholics. Cokeaholics, cakeaholics, pieaholics, burgeraholics, sugaraholics, junkfoodaholics and pizzaaholics anonymous

Many now boast, that they now longer drink water saying; "I can't drink plain water" but only consume sugar laden fizzy drinks and super sweet fruit juices, products that will only send their blood sugar levels haywire. Proper nutritious meals are too much hassle to prepare and when people are hungry they will eat snacks and confectionery, so snacks are regarded as food. As result the distinction between food and snacks has blurred, people will say "I need to get some food" and buy chocolate bars, crisps, as long as it can sate hunger, it is considered food.

Advertising now encourages us to keep our mouths moving constantly, from coffee to muffins to mints to chocolate bar to tea to sandwich to chewing gum to coffee to chewing gum to pizza to biscuit.

"In moderation" has been hurled through the plate glass window from ten stories up, crashed down onto the road and has been run over by a juggernaut truck carrying soft drinks to the nearest supermarket.

In developing countries, beef is still a treat and chicken rarer still, eaten on special occasions, but in industrialized nations, intensive farming methods have now made beef, pork, chicken and lamb, relatively cheap and common. Food processing methods have created cheap food in the form of burgers, pies, sausages, nuggets, kebabs and many other cheap mass produced, great tasting (salty),fat packed creations.

A large majority of people buy their main meal from takeaways, pizza, burgers, ready to eat chilled meals and frozen meals and restaurant fare. The older generation had the right attitude, all of the above meals were once in a while treats, once in a fucking blue moon, on special occasions, friday nights, an alternative, when you were genuinely too tired to cook or you had run out of ideas. You had it so rarely that when you did; you really appreciated and enjoyed it. Takeaway meals taste great, restaurants would go out of business if they did not but we now eat them so often that our taste buds have become dulled to their flavours, now its just another food product to be shovelled down our throats. When was the last time you appreciated a biriyani, with its spice combination of red chillies, coriander seeds, turmeric, cumin seeds, black pepper, garlic, ginger, cloves, cardamoms, star anise, cinnamon, bay leaves, mace and aromatic basmati rice? Or the delicate contrasts of crispy, sweet and sour pork, Hong Kong style served with fragrant jasmine rice, we are not just talking food but food to be appreciated and enjoyed. Aspects of another culture to be appreciated, now other cultures are just used as marketing gimmicks to sell more food, as a result we are sold a western version of food from India, china, Mexico, Thailand, America, Italy, morocco in the form of curries, stir fries, taco's, burgers, pizza and pasta to name a few.

Food manufacturers are seeking greater profits, consumers are looking to pay less for their food, the result of these two conflicting goals has made food cheaper, but manufacturers have used technological advances to create foods that will give them greater profit margins without a need to increase prices, as a result we have chicken bulked up with water, cattle fed with dead cows because they are cheap source of protein, sweetness added to everything because the price of sugar has fallen and abundantly grown subsidised corn can be turned into syrup, which is cheaper to transport because it is in liquid form and it also extends the shelf life of products, foods brought because they are expected to be tasty but they are actually salty, your bacon sandwich, can you actually taste the bacon or the salt. Food technology has not created superior or healthier products it has mainly allowed the food industry to extract extra value from existing products, nothing is allowed to go to waste, not even dead carcasses of cattle and sheep that appear in feed for cattle or chicken breasts with are injected with beef proteins allowing them to absorb large amounts of water, so as chicken is sold by weight, the companies are raking in a fortune selling water disguised as food to the public.

The cheaper the product, it will probably lack flavour of any kind but its main taste will be either be sweet or salty. For example the pack of economy frozen sausages brought for £1 which mainly tastes of salt, When you are eating that 99p burger can you taste the meat or the sugar in the ketchup, bread and salt in the burger?

Eat cheap: Die quick

The ingredients in food that is ruining our health are the additives like sugar, salt, fat, additives and preservatives added to make food more profitable for the manufacturers, these additives, increases our addition for junk food, These additives do not really need to be in our food supply, all they do is give food a longer shelf life, bulks up food, gives it colour, moisture and make it look attractive, Imagine the quality of our food, if all this crap was removed, the price of our food will increase but it would not kill us. The only benefit of cheap food is to the companies who make great profits selling it to us, for us; it ruins our health and shortens our lifespan.

All that money you think you are saving by buying cheap food, you won't live long enough to spend it.

This cheapening and degradation of food has no longer made food special, how much value and appreciation, are you going to place on a burger brought for 99p,or on a tin of baked beans that costs 13p.what is the nature and quality of the products in any tinned food that cost less that 25p?.

In the past if you wanted baked beans you brought Heinz or Crosse and Blackwell, and you had no problem with that. You did not shop around looking for a third alternative. Then improved manufacturing techniques that could produce a much cheaper and inferior tin of baked beans arrives, now you have the "basic value smart, better" range that nobody really asked for but is widely supplied and purchased. A result of the higher profit margins, cheap food conundrum.

I WANT IT ALL, I WANT IT NOW

People want more, so they get bigger portions, they want greater availability ,they want it now, they want it relatively cheap, as a result you fall over Kfc, MacDonald's, chilled meals, vending machines, frozen meals, Pizza hut, Wendy's, Burger king, Starbucks, Prêt a manger, Chinese takeaways, Indian takeaways, kebabs shops, sandwich bars, fish and chip shops, pub grub, petrol station snack stops, home delivery, quick bites, food on the good, food vans, snax stops, one minute in the microwave, free delivery, delivered piping hot or you get it free, free bottle of drink with your order, meat feast pizza with extra cheese, extra value meals, only 3,99,free poppadums with every order, buy one, get one free,99p menu,50% more, half price specials,10% more, value range, premium range, food programmes, only £1.99,food channels, celebrity chefs, more restaurants, more food magazines, more giveaways, recipe cards, magazine supplements, only £9.99 for the family bucket of salt drenched fried in oil chicken, constant food advertising. It never ends; all vying for attention and contributing to the non stop orgasmic feeding frenzy. As our food choices have expanded so has our waistlines.

Something's got to give
We overindulge
Our mouth never stops moving
We overeat,
Food manufacturers feed us more fatcrap
Aeroplanes have wider seats
Clothing retail outlets sell more large sizes
Car manufacturers make bigger cars
Drug manufacturers give us drugs to help counter the effects of our over weight bodies
Supermarkets provide us with bigger outlets; bigger

shopping trolleys and longer opening hours, so we can get our fatcrap fix 24 hours a day.
We get fat
Obesity creeps upon you slowly
We get all the health problems, obesity brings
We clog up the NHS, with our self inflicted diseases
We eat ourselves to death

Nuff said

Interlude

CHILDREN
They will not always do as you ask, they may even completely ignore your commands but they will unerringly copy what you do.
If you cannot cook
If you cannot stop eating crap
If you don't lead an active lifestyle
If you are on first name terms with you local takeaway restaurants
If you never walk anywhere
What do you expect your children to do.?
As a result of you inaction, they will not get to live as long as you.

Children have never been very good at listening to their elders, but they have never failed to imitate them.

James Baldwin

How much information has to be thrown at you before you decide to change your ways?
A word is enough for the wise

EVERY ACTION HAS A CONSEQUENCE

Decision;consequence

Ad astra per aspera

Willpower and discipline required for life

A moment on lips, a lifetime on the hips, waist, arm, thighs…

EAT LESS
MOVE MORE
CUT THE CRAP
EAT MORE FRUIT
EAT MORE VEGETABLES
KEEP AT IT

The only effective method to permanently lose weight

Live different

You need to get real; you will most likely have to give something up for the rest of your life, what will it be? Cakes? Biscuits? Fried foods?, fast food?, red meat? alcohol?, white flour?, the choice is yours. Weight maintenance is a lifetime commitment to lifestyle changes and as we all know, it is easier to lose excess weight than to keep it off.
On the other hand, you will definitely have to take up vigorous physical activity for the rest of your days.
If you cannot do it for yourself, do it for your children
The bible says *"Teach a child, the way to go and*

they will not depart from it"
Teach your child to eat and enjoy fruits, vegetables, good nutritious foods, once they get used to them, they are unlikely to change their habits when they get older. Unfortunately far too many parents give in to their children's demands and tantrums, as a reaction to this ghastly behaviour, they transform themselves into "best friends" and indulge their kids every whim. Now on the shopping trip, kids rule, the desire is only limited by their parent's budget and not their will.

As a result their tastes for sweet, salt and fatty foods are satisfied but their bodies are screaming for proper nutrition. As a result, we have children who have been fed up to their eyeballs with junk food but are nutrient, fibre, vitamin, and mineral deprived. Your child has junk for dinner and wakes up in the morning, looking like they have not slept for nights, gets to school, but still tired and unable to sleep, they are irritable, hyperactive and end up disturbing the classroom.

It is easy to see how a diet of fatcrap will handicap your child's mental and physical development.

Feeding your child with cheap, easy to purchase, prepare processed food means, you have devalued your child, a manufacturer mechanically reclaims chicken meat and skin, binds it with gums, adds various additives and sells it to you in the form of cheap chicken nuggets. Is the best you can do for the greatest unconditional love of your life? Don't you love them enough to spend time to make a healthy snack like a sandwich or to cook a great nutritious meal, of course not, no you cannot be bothered, you are far too busy watching television or chatting to your friends on the phone, so you reach for the nearest convenient alternative and feed that to you child. Does it make you feel proud? Is your child not worth the extra effort?

Child cruelty comes in many forms.

Most of our troubles stem from1 simple fact: we eat too fucking much!

Value for money?

Baked beans 17p
Frozen beef burgers 57p
Whole fresh chicken £2.75p
Bread 55p
Sliced ham £1.11p
Pack of frozen sausages £1.00
Meat pies 74p
Packet of pasta 30p
Value chicken nuggets £1.93p
Chicken burgers 94p
Fish fingers 85p
Frozen pizza £1.50
1.5 liter soft drink 17p
Buy one get one free
REALLY!

Real food costs more

There is nothing that is a more certain sign of insanity than to eat and drink the same crap, over and over and expect to live a long healthy life.

Effective living method
Refuse to have junk food in your house
Don't buy it
You won't eat it

Grow some backbone;fight the power

You will always face temptation, train yourself to eat

in moderation, eat smaller portions, eat at set times, if you eat chocolate bars everyday, gradually reduce your consumption to once or twice a week on scheduled days, the same for other fattening snacks, have a treat day, if you must but that does not give you permission to binge out.

Almost everybody knows the health implications of their food choices and eating habits, the message is getting through, people know they are eating themselves to death but carry on regardless. Why? They just cannot find within themselves the backbone, the intestinal fortitude to stick two fingers up to the adverts, the half price offers, the buy one get one free offers and say no thank you ,I really do not need, what you are offering.

Sometimes our health professionals are not in the best shape themselves, how many times has an overweight doctor or nurse, lectured you about not doing sufficient exercise or berated you for eating the wrong foods?

Decision;consequence

Everything you put in your mouth has a consequence on your body, it will either;

Be good for you, providing vitamins, nutrients and good calories

Or

It will be junk, it will be absolutely have no redeeming quality,

It will be full of empty calories, which do not have any nutritional value but will send your blood sugar level on a roller coaster ride, which over a prolonged period of time will lead to all kinds of health issues.

The greatest battle lies within

When it's all said and done, the fault lies not with the vast array of temptations put before you by the food industry and supermarkets. The final decision lies within yourself, nobody is forcing you to take your hard earned, overtaxed money and spend it on food that will ultimately ruin your health. despite all the advertising and marketing that seeks to persuade you to buy and consume, you are nobodies fool, It is time to engage your skepticism and look closely at the shit that's been shoveled your way.

You are not as gullible as the food industry thinks you are.

You have the power within you to make your own shopping list, go to the supermarket and leave with only the goods that were on your list. You have the power to walk past all the displays of new, reduced and special offer products, to get what you really need. It is time to exercise your will power.
After all you would never open the door to a known murderer, so why do let this silent, slow killer aka junk food, into your life?
Free your mind, exercise your willpower, it is possible.
Say to yourself:
I've got the power.

Then use it,

"No price is too high to pay for the privilege of owning yourself"

Nietzsche

It's not what we don't know; it's what we fail to do that makes us fat

The high cost of cheap food:

"Only after the last tree has been cut down

Only after the last river has been poisoned
Only after the last fish has been caught
Only then you will discover that money cannot be eaten"
Cree Indian prophecy
REPEAT AFTER ME
All things in moderation
All things in moderation
All things in moderation
All things in moderation
All things in moderation
All things in moderation
All things in moderation
All things in moderation
All things in moderation
All things in moderation
All things in moderation
All things in moderation
All things in moderation

Now live that truth.

Postscript

The microwave oven:the harbringer of the obesity epidemic
It has been said with the introduction of the microwave oven in the early 1980's into the kitchen has brought with it mass obesity. The entire chilled food industry could not exist without it. Before the mass introduction of the microwave oven most ready meals were frozen, that had to be heated in a conventional oven, so by the time you warmed up the oven, then reheated your meal to the required temperature, you realised that you were probably better off cooking your meal from scratch, after all you were not saving time. And if you had to cook,

then you were more likely to cook healthily.

So here comes a device that could reheat a meal in seconds or minutes, so at first, you used it to reheat left over's, you had cooked. Responding to the widespread use of microwave ovens in homes, food manufacturers brought out microwave meals, precooked chilled meals that could be reheated in minutes. Put the food in the microwave, by the time you set the table, food was piping hot ready. You no longer had time to wonder weather you were really hungry, when the hunger pangs hit you, now with microwave, the hunger impulse hits you and less than 5 minutes later you have sated that desire. All judgement ignored as there is no time lag between your hunger pangs and eventual satisfaction.

You don't have time to judge weather the food you are heating up is healthy, full of fibre or fattening, salt drenched. You just wolf it down. All the effort that has been made to produce food has been reduced to being heated and consumed in lest than 10 minutes. This hyper fast consumption has made us lose respect for our food and its sources and because it is so quick, it has made us consume more food quickly and that has made us obese.

There is no appreciation of the farmer's efforts or the beauty of Mother Nature. A farmer plants wheat, tends it and harvests it, it is transported to the miller who will turn grind the wheat into flour. It will then be shipped to the baker who will bake burger baps.

A cow is fed, looked after and reared for beef, a considerable amount of time and money is lavished on the animal. At the appropriate time, the animal is send to the abattoir, where it is slaughtered and then gets sent to the packing and processing factories were it is eventually turned into a beef patty.

The burger bap and burger are manufactured in a

chilled meal factory. When this creation finally reaches your kitchen, you put it in the microwave for 2 minutes and 5 minutes later, it has gone forever. You did not know and do not care to know about the chain that produced your food, it is any wonder that our relationship with food is entirely skewed.

In the future, with housing space at a premium, there will be no need for kitchens, just space for a sink, storage space, fridge freezer to store the frozen and chilled meals and a microwave.

I will do this no matter what it takes
I know no limitations
I will reach my destination

"I will get there"
Boys to Men

All things are possible,eat yourself to life

More from Perseverance Works.

The Winners Creed by Solicitus Civis
The winners creed on how to succeed after screwing up

This book is written for those of us, who have failed, messed up, screwed up, fallen and run from the field of battle, but on serious reflection have decided to get up ,dust ourselves off and enter the fray again. The Winners creed is the mindset you will need to adopt in order to succeed.
This book does not claim to have all the answers but is just trying to make you change your thinking and alter your mindset, because by changing the way you think, you will consequently change your life.
Now is time for you to change your life, it is up to you to take control of your destiny, as it has been said if anything is going to be, it is up to you.
It is time for you to decide that no matter what the politician's do, what the economy does, you must decide your own destiny, so when you are on your death bed, old and grey, the only tune you should be singing is Frank Sinatra's "My way".

Available to order from lulu.com

Kitchen Safety Record

Created by Culina Salus
Kitchen daily diary refill sheets are no longer sent out by the Food Standards Agency.

Don't waste money photocopying or using up expensive printer ink or looking unprofessional with pieces of paper. Get the replacement now:

Kitchen Safety Record Created by Culina Salus

Contains:

- ➢ **Daily dairy sheets**
- ➢ **Temperature records**
- ➢ **Contacts list**
- ➢ **Cleaning schedule**
- ➢ **Staff training record**
- ➢ **Supplier list**

The daily diary sheet also incorporates the fridge temperature records, so you only need to record all information on one sheet.

Recommended for **ALL** kitchens including Hotels, Restaurants, Schools, Colleges, Hospitals, Nursing homes, Takeaways, Cafes, Mobile catering vans, Home caterers, Church and Community halls-*wherever food is prepared for members of the public.*

- ➢ *Order now at* **Amazon.co.uk** *by entering:kitchen safety record or culina salus into the search box.*

Culina Salus,a veteran of the catering industry with decades of extensive experience as a chef,chef and catering manager, event caterer ,food safety trainer working for companies such as Hilton

Hotel, The BBC, Camberwell college of Arts, Tropical dream village in Malindi Kenya, Scolarest and Compass catering

> **Abide by Food Safety Regulations, keep safe and legally compliant, get your copy now at Amazon.co.uk by entering:** *kitchen safety record* **or** *culina salus* **into the search box.**

Safe food depends on a hygienic and well managed kitchen

Available to order from Amazon.co.uk

www.ingramcontent.com/pod-product-compliance
Lightning Source LLC
Chambersburg PA
CBHW060218290526
45789CB00003B/1316